Be a Fat-Burning Machine

The Metabolism Advantage

[RS Johnson]

Table of Contents

Introduction

The weight-loss industry has become so flooded with "experts" and "breakthrough" products that it's nearly impossible to know how to lose weight successfully any longer. Almost every week, a new "miracle" is promoted by daytime TV shows and the internet. As long as trillions of dollars are in the weight loss industry, opportunistic companies will devise new ways to use our money properly.

Weight-loss propaganda can be identified by the use of words like "groundbreaking," "advanced formula," and "clinically proven," which are marketing terms used to trick us into parting with more of our hard-earned money in exchange for simple solutions to our expanding waistlines.

Unfortunately, their methods are perfectly legal as well. In addition, there are some excellent weight-loss programs available, as well as a few high-quality products. Still, for the most part, the industry is full of unsubstantiated hype and false claims designed to provide various businesses with a piece of the billion-dollar weight-loss pie.

No such thing as a magical product exists. Weight-loss solutions aren't found in some magical elixir derived from a rare fruit that only grows on a Tibetan mountaintop.

Obesity is on the rise, and there is no end in sight because humans have strayed from eating foods compatible with our genetic programming. We are properly designed to eat foods that our bodies recognize and contain nutrients that we can quickly assimilate. When we don't, we get hormonal imbalances, a slower metabolism, and more fat storage.

The Dangers in Losing Weight

When it comes to losing weight, almost everyone relies on calorie counting. We weigh our food, download smartphone apps, and become Rain Man at math, all in the name of staying within caloric boundaries and losing X number of pounds per week.

Eating fewer calories than exercising can result in weight loss; however, this isn't a healthy method. This is because we frequently do not change what we eat. Instead, we try to eat less.

Rather than eating more fruits and vegetables, leafy greens, fish, and other natural foods (which nourish our cells), we end up buying "low-calorie" items at fast-food restaurants and attempting to eat fewer hamburgers, less pasta, and fewer cookies, all while restricting ourselves more and more until we reach our target weight.

Losing weight is meaningless if you end up destroying your health in the process. Unfortunately, there are a lot of skinny, sick people out there.

Obesity does contribute to disease. However, the same unhealthy lifestyle that contributes to obesity also contributes to illness. Therefore, our efforts to lose weight for health reasons will be futile unless we change the lifestyle that has led to our obesity.

To truly succeed, we must balance our desire to be thin with our desire to be healthy.

The Hormonal Reasons We Gain Weight

The loss of weight is not counting calories, drinking protein shakes or chemical shakes, or seeking the perfect treatment or program. Instead, the amount of fat around your middle, as well as the ease with which you lose it, is entirely determined by your hormone levels (specific insulin).

The more insulin you have, the more fat you will store and the heavier you will become. Two factors cause high insulin levels:

- Eating high sugar/high carbohydrate foods.

- Overeating of them at one time.

Here's how it works: Your body uses the food you eat to nourish cells and generate energy. If you take more than you want at once, your blood glucose will rise, and you release insulin to store the excess glycogen in your liver and muscles (for energy). However, those stockpiles quickly fill up, and once complete, the remainder is stockpiled as fat.

The worst offenders for raising insulin levels (and thus causing fat storage) are:

Carbohydrates that have been processed include grains, pasta, bread, bagels, snack bars, crackers, and cereal. In addition, sugar, artificial sweeteners, food chemicals, and snack foods such as soda, cookies, chips, baked goods, and pastries are all bad for you.

Sugar-free foods will still cause weight gain because they are typically high in carbohydrates and other synthetic chemicals and additives that slow metabolism.

Other packaged foods in wrappers, bags, and boxes are all the foods found in fast-food restaurants and grocery store aisles, including those marketed as "low-calorie" or "zero-calories." More on that in a moment.

Our cells become insulin resistant as we repeatedly raise our insulin levels through overeating and poor dietary choices. This is not an error but a protective mechanism.

Overweight people develop type 2 diabetes, high blood pressure, and high cholesterol due to their diet, not because they are overweight. Another side effect is a decrease in the production of "satiety" hormones, which tell us when we are full.

People with type 2 diabetes may believe that their insulin levels are too low and must take insulin orally or by injection, but this is not the case. Instead, insulin resistance has developed in type 2 diabetics, requiring more insulin to perform the same function as before. If the proper guidelines are followed, both type 2 diabetes and insulin resistance can be reversed.

When insulin levels remain high due to high carbohydrate and sugar intake over time, fat cells become insulin resistant, making it nearly impossible for the body to burn fat for energy. This destroys your ability to lose weight regardless of caloric restriction or exercise commitment.

Chapter 1 | Weight Loss Myths That Should Just Die Already

Let us be precise. We don't want to lose weight. We want to lose weight. Essentially, we want to feel better about ourselves and look good without our clothes on. However, simply losing weight will not achieve this. You can starve yourself and lose 10 pounds, but if you achieve your goal through deprivation, you will also lose muscle and may still be unable to fit into those high school jeans.

Let's dispel some tired fat-loss myths that should have died a long time ago.

Fat Loss Myth #1 – Eating Fat Makes You Fat

If fat caused people to gain weight, everyone on a low-fat diet would be thin, but they aren't. Every food product on supermarket shelves appears to be low-fat, fat-free, or low-calorie, but this does not solve our obesity problem.

When fat or calories are removed, chemicals and fake sugars are added, and these chemicals disrupt our hormone balance, metabolism, and health.

When high cholesterol became a problem, doctors advised us to avoid eating fat. However, people needed to eat SOMETHING, so we resorted to processed carbohydrates.

Pasta, bread, rice, and cereal (processed foods in wrappers, bags, and boxes) became the staples of the average American Diet. Since then, we've only grown larger and sicker, and the trend is only getting worse.

Eating more HEALTHY fat and less sugar, carbs, and grains will assist you in losing fat. If sugar is not burned for energy, the body burns fat and loses weight easily.

Fat Loss Myth #2 – I Just Need To Exercise More

Simply put, you can't outrun your fork. We get toned and strong at the gym. We lose weight in the kitchen.

First, just because you burn off some extra calories through exercise does not negate the negative health effects of junk food. Second, limiting calories and increasing exercise results in long-term weight loss only for the most committed dieters. This is because the body will eventually fight back against deprivation (starvation) by clinging to the food you eat for dear life.

People who do this frequently express their frustration by saying, "I just can't seem to lose these last ten pounds."

Weight loss has little to do with the number of calories you consume or expend. However, it has everything to do with the TYPES of food you eat and how they affect your body. When you eat real food, there is little need for calorie restriction.

Fat Loss Myth #3 – It's Genetic

The medical community has persuaded us that the human body is frail and genetically predisposed to illness. This is completely false!

Because the advice we've been getting for health and weight loss for the last 40 years has been WRONG, the old stand-by response became, "Well, it's genetic, and there's nothing you can do." Unfortunately, this keeps us all trapped in the medical hamster wheel of chronic disease, prescription medication, and surgery to solve our health problems.

There isn't a single insect, plant, or animal on the planet that passes on the degenerative disease to its offspring. We may be born to certain illnesses, but the right lifestyle will not activate those genes. Only .01 percent of diseases are classified as genetic, and obesity is not one of them.

The majority of people who believe their weight problems are genetic are simply misinformed. This can be deeply annoying when all conventional wisdom says you have to lose weight and still have no results.

When it comes to weight issues, many factors come into play, such as stress, sleep patterns, prescription drugs, exercise routines, and, of course, diet, but the body is genetically programmed to be lean, muscular, and strong. So if yours isn't, the issue is most likely NOT your genes, but rather the lifestyle signals you send them.

The Most Important Fat Loss Myth

Despite all of the commercials, gimmicks, and neighbors

selling MLM weight-loss supplements, you can't avoid nature.

The body is programmed to follow certain rules, and breaking them for an extended period can have serious consequences. You can certainly deceive the body for a while, which is why many programs and fads work at first (or at least until the auto-ship program triggers another sale and charges your credit card), but the body eventually catches up with you.

Chapter 2 | Why Diet Foods Make You Gain Weight

Monica was about 45 pounds overweight when I first met her. She'd tried every gimmick and program under the sun in an attempt to get back into her skinny jeans, but nothing worked. She assumed that her metabolism was slowing down with age, her body composition was changing, and she had a thyroid problem or needed more exercise, but nothing she tried helped her reach her goal.

Monica also had a fat-free food cabinet, a desk drawer full of "all-natural" diet bars, a freezer full of "healthy, low-calorie" frozen dinners, and she spent an hour on the treadmill every day to avoid exceeding her 1,500 calorie limit, not realizing that all of this was contributing to her weight problem.

These are several reasons why dietary foods undermine your efforts to reduce weight loss:

Diet-Food Ingredients That Make You Gain Weight.

Diet foods contain hidden chemicals that almost certainly contribute to weight gain. But, unfortunately, they're cleverly disguised, so you're less likely to find out about them.

If it's processed, canned, comes in a box, is purchased through a window, or is labeled low-fat or low-calorie, it almost certainly contains MSG. MSG is also known as yeast extract and hydrolyzed protein (among other things), and it is almost certainly present whenever you see:

- Gelatin
- Protein Isolates
- Soy Protein
- Whey Protein
- Carrageenan
- Citric Acid
- Maltodextrin
- Flavorings
- Others

MSG makes fake food taste authentic. If you find it in food, it means the product isn't fresh and contains synthetic ingredients. For example, fast food restaurants use this method to make fake turkey, chicken, and beef taste real meat.

Why MSG Makes You Gain Weight?

MSG is a neurotoxin, which means it interferes with brain and nervous system function. For example, have you ever noticed that an hour after eating Chinese food, you're hungry again, or that "you can't eat just one" when it comes to that bag of chips? This is because MSG messes with your brain's receptors, preventing you from feeling full. This way, you can eat until the bag is empty, at which point you'll have to buy more.

MSG is also addictive, which is why it is found in most

foods in wrappers, bags, and boxes. What food company wouldn't want you to become addicted to their products?

Do you ever wonder how researchers conduct obesity experiments on laboratory rats? They don't go out and look for obese rats. There aren't any. They must MAKE them obese, which they do by feeding them MSG. MSG causes an increase in insulin levels (in rats and humans), which causes the body (in rats and humans) to store fat.

The phrase "zero calories" is a deception. However, a labeling loophole allows this term to be used even though it is false. Because artificial sugars do not exist in nature, the body does not produce enzymes to metabolize them. This is how they can put a big fat ZERO in the calories column.

When sugar enters the liver, it decides whether to store it, burn it, or convert it to fat. However, it has been demonstrated that artificial sugar bypasses this process and converts directly to fat.

Trans Fats

These are unnatural fats found in almost any diet food (look for hydrogenated oils). However, researchers have shown Trans-fats to cause a redistribution of fat cells to the abdomen and increase body weight even when dietary calories are controlled.

So when all the other factors are equal, the person who uses trans-fats (diet or processed foods) gets more weight if two people eat the same calories.

Chapter 3 | Reasons Why Your Weight Loss Efforts Have Stalled

When hormone levels are balanced, it is natural to have vibrant health, a strong build, and easy weight management. However, numerous lifestyle factors can impact our hormones and prevent us from reaching our goals.

Below are amongst the most likely reasons for a weight loss plateau::

- As we discussed in the previous chapter, you may be eating too many diet foods. Diet foods are designed to be low-calorie or fat-free because food manufacturers understand that you will most likely purchase products based on these characteristics. However, they don't tell you that when calories and fat are removed, fake sugars and other chemicals take their place, causing hormone levels to shift, metabolism to slow, and the body to store fat at a faster rate.

- You are consuming insufficient calories. Calorie counters believe that if restricting calories help them lose weight, restricting a large number of calories will help them lose more weight faster. But, unfortunately, the body perceives severe calorie restriction as starvation and will eventually turn against you, fighting for dear life to retain the calories you consume.

- You're overdoing it on the cardio. Weight loss is not guaranteed simply because you spend an hour every day on the treadmill. Long cardio sessions can work against you. Because your body interprets exercise as stress, stress causes the release of a hormone called cortisol, which breaks down energy reserves for immediate use. This reaction is healthy and natural in the short term, but prolonged cortisol increases eventually lead to insulin resistance, bone density loss, loss of lean muscle mass, and weight gain.

Short bursts (10-15 minutes) of high-intensity training (like sprints, plyometrics, and bodyweight exercise) have been shown in studies to increase the fat-burning potential of muscle, improve the efficiency with which the body burns fat, and be a more time-efficient strategy for fat burning exercise.

- You're under a lot of pressure. Every type of stress triggers the "fight or flight" response (physical, emotional, or chemical). This stress response causes changes in hormone levels as the body shuts down all processes that are not immediately necessary for survival. But, again, this is completely normal unless the stress is chronic, in which case it leads to increased fat storage around the belly and decreases thyroid function.

- You're not getting enough fat in your diet. It might appear counterintuitive, but you must consume more fat if you want to lose fat. First, however, we must distinguish between healthy and unhealthy fat. Trans fats, omega-6 fats, and processed fats are examples of unhealthy fats found in processed foods. Healthy fats, on the other hand (fats found in fish, organ meats, nuts, coconut, eggs, avocados, olives, and so on) are required for proper cellular function.

Contrary to popular belief, healthy fats do not result in weight gain or higher cholesterol levels.

Consumption of healthy fats rather than sugar gives us energy, maintains us satiated for longer periods, and causes the body to combust with fat.

- You aren't getting enough rest. Sleep deprivation is an often overlooked source of health problems. This is because our sleep patterns have a significant impact on our hormone levels. We gain weight due to poor sleeping habits because the greatest surge in fat-burning hormones occurs during deep sleep.

- You consume an excessive amount of carbohydrates. The standard American Diet (SAD) contains many processed carbohydrates, which mess with your blood sugar and insulin levels. As a result, fat cells become insulin resistant over time, making it nearly impossible for the body to burn fat regardless of how much you exercise or how few calories you consume.

Chapter 4 | Turn Your Body Into a Fat-Burning Machine

You can transform your body into a fat-burning machine by adopting the right lifestyle. There are no shakes, pills, or programs required; simply the right information and the desire to follow it. It's not even that difficult.

Products designed to assist you in losing weight are typically either unsustainable or unhealthy. Crash diets and toxic protein powders do nothing but drain your bank account and leave you heavier than when you started. Physiological reasons exist, but you gain back more weight than yourself if you use these gimmicks for another article.

How Your Genes Adapt to Your Diet?

Almost every physical limitation in human life is blamed on our genes. But, unfortunately, it's an easy way out that requires little explanation and keeps us trapped in our disease-care system based on "symptom relief."

Cancer? It's in your blood. There is nothing you can do. What is the cause of heart disease? It's inherited. Thank you to your parents. Diabetes? Do you have high cholesterol? Osteoporosis? Do you have a bad back? Genes, genes, genes, genes, but don't worry; there are plenty of expensive drugs you can take for the rest of your life to compensate.

Our genes do play a role in our weight, but probably not in the way you think. Some strange error does not cause obesity in your DNA that was passed down from your parents. Instead, being overweight is the result of living a life that contradicts our genetic programming.

Are You Sugar Adapted?

If you eat a typical American diet high in processed carbohydrates, soda, and artificial sugar (foods in wrappers, bags, and boxes), your genes will alter how your body processes food.

In effect, you become "sugar-adapted," which means you teach your body to burn sugar (glucose) for fuel because it is always available.

Every glucose (sugar) is converted into glucose during digestion, which increases the level of insulin. Insulin is the hormone that is in charge of storing excess sugar as fat. Therefore, the higher your blood sugar, the higher your insulin levels will be, and the more fat you store.

Sugar-addicted people are typically overweight, have noticeable periods of fatigue during the day, and frequently experience cravings for comfort foods or foods that are emotionally appealing. They struggle with dieting because calorie counting always leaves them hungry. They are not satisfied with vegetables and fruits. They believe that eating a salad for dinner isn't "real food" and that they need something "heavier" or they'll "starve" for the rest of the night.

How does being sugar-adapted make you overweight?

Because the body has learned to use sugar as its primary energy source, hunger will return once insulin has cleared glucose from the bloodstream.

A sugar-adapted dieter's body will not only retain the calories consumed, but it will also be more likely to store fat AND make you crave more sugar and carbs shortly after eating.

Become a Fat-Burning Machine

The key to becoming a fat-burning machine is to train your body to use fat as fuel rather than sugar. Because our genes are already hardwired in this manner, this can be accomplished relatively quickly and easily.

Fat-adapted people maintain their weight effortlessly. They are less hungry, stay satiated for longer periods after eating, and have plenty of energy. They have few sugar cravings and instead crave their favorite nutrient-dense snacks. Even when sugar and carbs are consumed in excess, their bodies handle them efficiently and resist fat storage.

So, how exactly do you become fat-adapted? By reducing your intake of sugar, carbs, and grains while increasing your intake of HEALTHY fats. When blood sugar levels are low, insulin levels remain low. There is no fat storage if insulin levels remain low. The body turns to fat if there is no burnt sugar for fuel. In short, you're "adapted to fat."

Please remember that you should not stock your pantry with processed junk marketed as "low-carb" diet foods. These items are devoid of nutrition and are laced with harmful chemicals.

Also, when you see the words "low-fat" or "fat-free" on a label, think CARB-BOMB! This is because sugar replaces fat when it is removed.

Best Food Choices for Reprogramming Your Genes

It may sound strange, but you must eat more fat while limiting carbohydrates if you want to become fat-adapted. Those fats, of course, should be healthy, fats found naturally in real food.

Organ meats, beef, poultry, eggs, nuts (macadamia, walnuts, hazelnuts, almonds, pecans), seeds, coconut and coconut oil, olives avocados, and olive oil, and fatty fish (tuna, mackerel, herring, trout, sardines, and salmon) should all be included in your diet regularly.

Those aren't the only food you should eat. But you will only be sabotage by trying to remove fat from your diet. So instead, make sure you're getting plenty of leafy green vegetables and low-sugar fruits like berries, stone fruits, lemons, and limes.

Chapter 5 | The Basics of the Real Food Diet

The key to losing weight and keeping it off is to eat natural foods. If it grows from a tree or a plant or is something that humans can typically hunt down, the body will recognize it.

Because apples are made of the same material as humans, your body knows exactly what to do with them. A cupcake, on the other hand, is a different story.

Fake food, also known as food in wrappers, bags, and boxes, is manufactured in a factory and DOES NOT contain nutrients that the body recognizes. As a result, we don't process them well, and our bodies react to them as toxins.

This is not conducive to a slim waistline or a healthy body.

5 Essential Steps to a Real Food Diet

Our goal should be to consume 90 percent of our calories from whole foods. This means that 90% of our food choices should be whole, organic, and unprocessed. We keep the other 10% for fun and when we can't eat real food (travel, social functions, etc.).

On the other hand, a transition from Standard US Diet (SAD) to a 90/10 diet can be difficult. Carbohydrates and sugar, the SAD's mainstay, have been scientifically proven to be as addictive as cocaine, making breaking the SAD habit difficult and unpleasant for some.

Epigenetic changes result in unconscionably high energy, efficient weight management, and overall health due to a real dieting low in carbohydrates and sugar.

Unless you're not one of those people who can change their lives completely in one day, here's the best way to progressively move into a real diet.

Step 1: The Purge

This is the first concept I teach to anyone who wants to change their life through nutrition. However, because it is so drastic, not everyone can pull it off. If you cannot complete the purge, begin with the "half-purge," as described below.

The purge entails going through your cupboards and pantry and discarding all processed food in wrappers, bags, and boxes. It's not real food if it doesn't rot eventually. Bread (yes, even whole grain), pasta, bagels, breakfast & snack bars, cereal, chips, crackers, microwave popcorn, and other phony foods are examples.

The refrigerator/freezer must also be dismantled. Ice cream, frozen dinners, frozen pizzas, waffles, microwaveable breakfast sandwiches, and similar items.

You can't eat it if it's not in your house, and if you're serious about changing your body and your health, the purge must occur at some point.

If you have an uncontrollable desire for your favorite snack, force yourself to leave the house to get it. Even so, only buy enough for one sitting, not for five days.

The Half-Purge

If you think the purge is too drastic, the half-purge is a much easier option and should be your first step. But, first, make a list of everything in your cupboards, pantry, and refrigerator (especially anything processed) that you could live without eating for the rest of your life and not mind, and start with those.

Step 2: Add More Real Food

If you're making a gradual transition to a real food diet, don't start by putting yourself through agonizing deprivation. The prospect of never again eating the foods you enjoy is often the most frightening of all, followed by some all-too-common excuses:
"I want to have fun with my life." "Everything in moderation," as the saying goes. "Food is meant to be enjoyed."
And to these I reply...
"It is more enjoyable to be disease-free than to please your taste buds for a few seconds."
"Everything in moderation" is a phrase used by those who are not fully committed to changing their ways.
"Healthy food CAN taste delicious."
There are no excuses when you're truly ready to eat differently and lose weight. However, step 2 does not require you to give up your favorite foods just yet. Instead, start eating more real food (particularly leafy greens) at each meal. If fruits and vegetables make up 0-25 percent of your plate, try increasing it a little each day. You eventually want your entire plate to be made up of whole, unprocessed foods grown by the Earth.

Step 3: Begin Limiting Carbohydrates

It is not unusual for someone following the SAD to consume more than 300 grams of processed carbohydrates per day. As a result, obesity and various diseases such as cancer, insulin resistance, type 2 diabetes, thyroid issues, high cholesterol, osteoporosis, heart disease, rapid aging, and many others result from this excessive carbohydrate intake.

If you're going to count something, start with carbs rather than calories.

Most people require 100-150 grams of TOTAL carbs per day to maintain their weight. That amount should be reduced to 50-100 grams for weight loss. 20-50 grams of total carbohydrates per day is ideal for rapid weight loss and disease reversal.

Remember to get your carbs from fruits and vegetables rather than cereal and bread.

Expect intense sugar cravings, severe energy fluctuations, and other strange symptoms (often referred to as the "low-carb flu") during this phase. It typically takes a few days or several weeks to burn fat for fuel rather than sugar through your body switch gears.

Step 4: Find Healthy Snacks

SAD eaters are voracious smackers. They consume soda regularly, snack on chips and popcorn while watching TV, and have a sweet dessert after dinner. They sometimes skip dinner entirely and go straight for the dessert!

During the day, it is simple to avoid junk food. But,

unfortunately, people tend to slip after their evening meal. So keep healthy, whole-food snacks on hand at all times.

Vegetables and hummus, apples and almond butter, berries and Greek yogurt, and leftovers from your real food dinner are also options.

Step 5: Start Cooking at Home

The most common reason for not cooking at home is a lack of time. They are so preoccupied with life, work, and family that spending an hour in the kitchen every night is simply not an option.

Although a lack of time is the most common excuse, failure to plan is the most common reason. When you're tired and hungry, you're much more likely to a drive-through or throw a frozen pizza in the oven if you're not prepared, but it takes the same amount of time to cook a chicken breast and a side of asparagus as it does a frozen pizza.

Planning is essential when you have a career and/or children who participate in sports and other activities, so prioritize daily meals as if they were as important as everything else. The key is to keep matters as easy as you can.

Chapter 6 | diet Hacks to Keep Weight Loss On Track

The diet industry believes we are illiterate. They show it every day, by the way, with headlines such as: "Lose Belly Fat Like Crazy with this One Simple Trick." There are also commercials promising six-pack abs without diet or workout, with fitness models claiming to be just like you, mentioning "clinical trials," which we will never see.

And you can get it all for nothing!!! "Ahem, just pay shipping and processing on our auto-ship program."

On the other hand, such advertisements draw attention and generate sales, so they are unlikely to go away anytime soon.

The #1 Way to Lose Weight

This next sentence, if you can get it into your head, will change your life forever... Ready? I've said it before...

Getting healthy is the most effective way to lose weight.

At the end of the story, getting healthy (and thus losing weight) necessitates changing what we put in our mouths rather than simply eating less. It necessitates a lifestyle change and commitment that lasts long after the desire to fit into our skinny jeans has faded.

Even if you've made a firm commitment to yourself, most people find that the change process is a long one, with many setbacks and blunders along the way until a new way of life In order to assist you keep track of your life and health, there are here a couple of diet hacks. In this respect.

Please be aware that it is not a 10 pounds loss guide in ten days. If you're still considering such ideas, you're not serious about healthily losing weight.

Don't keep food that you try to avoid in your house

You can avoid many common pitfalls if you force yourself to get up, put on your shoes, and drive to the grocery store every time you crave sugar, treats, or junk food. This way, there are numerous points between your house and the store where you can rest.

Perhaps it will be too cold to go out, perhaps you will not have the $10 to spend, or perhaps you will suddenly find some self-control, but it will be much more difficult to change your mind if the junk is only a few feet away.

If you have to travel, but only one service. You're going to eat, and then it's going to be gone... no more tomorrow. Make yourself go for a walk or do push-ups before you leave to add another layer of security.

Eat something good before eating something bad.

This works for kids, so it should work for adults as well. Make it a rule that if you want a cookie, you must first eat an apple. If you want a soda, you must first drink 8 ounces of water. When you do this, two things will happen:

Sometimes you won't eat anything at all.

Other times, you're going to eat junk, but you're going to be stuffed with fruit (or anything else) and will not eat over.

When you're hungry, eat healthy foods you love.

If you like omelets, pistachios, smoothies, vegetable stir-fry, chicken kabobs, apples with almond butter, and so on, eat these instead of junk food when you get hungry, whether it's 11 a.m. or 9 p.m. Choose real food from a box or sack if you want your palate buds to satisfy.

Remove and not care for any food you can go without.

Also referred to as the "half-purge."

You may not be hungry for a bowl of fried shrimp and Lucky Charms, but if you're desperate enough, you'll eat one (just ask my college roommate). If you're going to cheat, make it count by satisfying your craving rather than reaching for anything because you're bored.

Change one thing at a time.

Don't try to change your entire diet in a single day. Such an approach is rarely successful. Instead, concentrate on making one small change at a time. Begin with the simple adjustments and work your way up to the more difficult ones.

1. Don't reward yourself with food.

You're not a dog, so don't treat yourself after a few successful days. If you have such a relationship with food, you will never achieve your objectives. Rather, make your reward health, vitality, and long life.

2. Keep a food diary.

This is not for calorie, carb, or carrot stick counting. It is intended to keep you informed about your choices. So make a list of everything you eat BEFORE you eat it.

This will give you a chance to pause and think about what you're about to do, as well as a chance to change your mind.

3. Watch yourself eat.

This technique, while cruel and unusual at times, works. Eat all of your meals while naked (or in your underwear) in front of a full-length mirror. The majority of us are unconcerned about how we chew, swallow, and generally consume our food. This practice will quickly make you aware and keep you mindful of every bite.

4. Eat protein and healthy fat rather than carbs.

Your body begins to produce an appetite suppressant when you put food in your mouth.

Carbohydrates cause the least amount of appetite suppressants to be released. Therefore, protein is the most abundant, followed by healthy fat. This is why you feel hungry after eating a banana but not after eating a steak.

5. Plan ahead.

This accounts for 80% of your success or failure. The willingness to plan often distinguishes those who slip from those who do not. For example, if you haven't prepared for lunch, you're more likely to make a poor choice when your stomach grumbles. Instead, you'll go to the drive-through or the vending machine because you're "starving."

If you already have something healthy on hand, you'll have to come up with another reason to eat that Snickers bar.

Chapter 7| Do Weight Loss Shakes and Supplements Work?

In our search for easy weight-loss solutions, the leagues of desperate people are looking for the right supplement or shake to magically give them the edge they need to succeed in losing weight. So let me make one thing clear...

There is ZERO scientific evidence that ANY weight-loss supplement or shake can boost your metabolism, block fat absorption, or make any other purely speculative marketing claim.

Believe me, and there is no need for magic or miracles if you follow the advice in this eBook. However, the food you're genetically programmed to eat contains magic and miracles.

If you incorporate a supplement or shake into your weight-loss efforts, it should be used ONLY to nourish your cells while you transition to a healthy lifestyle and 90/10 real food diet. They should NOT be used to restrict calories or alter body processes in any way.

Preservatives, colorings, fillers, GMOs, artificial sugars, flavorings, and artificial fiber.

When our clients ask, we recommend a few such products. They are as follows:

- Raw Protein
- Perfect Weight Multi
- Raw Fit

After a thorough search, we also discovered a suitable "grab and go" snack bar made with truly all-natural ingredients and organic nuts.

Conclusion

If you believe that any extra calories you consume, go straight to your belly or thighs, you do not imagine things. Instead, your genes, hormones, age, lifestyle, and other factors are usually the areas where you store fat.

To keep you alive and safe, your body stores calories as fat. The challenge is figuring out how to get rid of that excess fat.

Fat-burning gimmicks like working out in the fat-burning zone, spot reduction, and foods or supplements that supposedly burn more fat are all popular. Learn to use a variety of practice methods to burn fat instead.

Visit And Buy the Other Books of This Author

Happy Saint Patrick's Day: Saint Patrick's Day Planner/Journal with 8.5x11 inches and 100 Pages

https://www.amazon.com/dp/B09BY841SZ

St. Patrick's Day: Saint Patrick's Day Planner/Journal with 8.5x11 inches and 100 Pages

https://www.amazon.com/dp/B09BY7XWGD

Happy Easter: Easter Egg Patterns Worksheet: 8.5x11 Inches 60 Pages

https://www.amazon.com/dp/B09BT2B6F3

Easter Hunt Activity Happy Easter: Easter Hunt Activity Journal | Notebook size 8.5x11 60 Pages

https://www.amazon.com/dp/B09BY7XWKL

Easter Day Spring Writing Assignment worksheet: Easter Day Spring Writing Assignment worksheet | 8.5x11 60 Pages | Spring Worksheet

https://www.amazon.com/dp/B09BY5HNVB

Cinco De Mayo: Large Updated Organizer with Daily Spreads For 2 Months with Cover Paperback https://www.amazon.com/dp/B09BY8178L

Taking full charge of your finance: Easy Guide to Personal Finance

https://www.amazon.com/Taking-full-charge-your-finance/dp/B099C8S85Z

Sure, Steps to Wealth Creation: How to Build Wealth from Nothing

https://www.amazon.com/Sure-Steps-Wealth-Creation-Nothing/dp/B099C3GNQH

All You Need to Know About Cryptocurrency: Understanding Risk and Reward in Investing

https://www.amazon.com/Need-Know-About-Cryptocurrency-Understanding/dp/B099C3GNML

Eliminating Your Debt in 12 (x) Easy Steps and Keep Them Off: A Practical Guide to Eliminating Your Debt Forever!

https://www.amazon.com/Eliminating-Your-Debt-Easy-Steps/dp/B099BZX4FX

NLP For Beginners

https://www.amazon.com/NLP-Beginners-RS-Johnson-ebook/dp/B098JBH28Q

Credit Repair Secrets

<-END->